100%WAYS TO STAY HEALTHY WITH MORINGA

Moringa (The Magic Tree)

I0503591

Dr.BAYO

TABLE OF CONTENTS

Introduction

Moringa is a tree that has been used for years in India for every of their food, to building materials, and also for its beneficial properties. This 'miracle tree' truly is wondrous in that each part of the tree is helpful. The roots, stems, leaves, seed pods, resin and flowers are considered to be healing herbs in Ayurvedic (traditional Indian curing system) and Unani (traditional Middle Eastern curing system) folk medicine. In modern times, the leaves and seed pods are made used extensively because of their nutrient content and modern reseaches are investigating their numerous potential.

Moringa is native to the sub Himalayan mountain region mostly in India and has been knowned to southwest Asia, southwest and northeast Africa, Madagascar, the Philippines, and in the United States in California, Arizona, Hawaii and Florida. This tree is in the Moringaceae, or horseradish tree, family which is very related to the papaya containing Caricaceae family. It is the one genus, comprises thirteen species one such species being M. stenopetala, a species native to and planted in Africa.

The generic name is obtained from the Tamil (language spoken in southern India and northeast Sri Lanka) word 'murungai' meaning twisted pod. And 'oleifera' is Latin meaning 'oil-bearing' because of the seeds high oil content.

Moringa is drought tolerant and thrives in semi-arid, tropical, and subtropical climates and is one of the highest commonly planted food plants in the world. It is cultivated in India, Pakistan, Africa, the Philippines, and the Caribbean. Moreso, it is planted in numerous countries in Central and South America due to it's easy grow and has an increase market potential, therefore potentially providing an alternative to deforestation. It is also planted richly in African countries to cater for their Own malnourished populations

Chapter One

WHAT IS MORINGA?

Moringa is a plant that is known to areas of India, Pakistan, Bangladesh, and Afghanistan. It is also cultivated in the tropics. The leaves, bark, flowers, fruit, seeds, and root are used for medicine.

Moringa is used for "tired blood" (anemia), arthritis and other joint
pain (rheumatism), asthma, cancer, constipation, diabetes
, diarrhea, seizures, stomach pain, stomach and intestinal ulcers, intestinal spasms, headache, heart problems, high blood pressure, kidney stones, symptoms
of menopause, thyroid disorders, and infections.

Moringa is also used to decrease swelling, as an antioxidant, to stop spasms, increase sex drive (as an aphrodisiac), stop pregnancy, boost the immune system, and increase breast milk production. Some people take it as a nutritional supplement or tonic. It is also taken as a "water pill" (diuretic).

Moringa is sometimes robbed directly to the skin as a germ-killer or drying agent (astringent). It is also robbed to the skin for treating pockets of infection (abscesses), athlete's foot, dandruff, gum
disease (gingivitis), snakebites, warts, and wounds.

Oil derived from moringa seeds are used in foods, perfume, and hair care products, and as a machine lubricant.

Moringa is a vital food source in various parts of the world. Because it can be cultivated cheaply and easily, and the leaves contain lots of vitamins and minerals when dried, moringa is helpful in India and Africa in feeding programs to fight against malnutrition. The immature green pods (drumsticks) are cooked similarly to green beans, while the seeds are removed from more mature pods and prepared like peas or roasted like nuts. The leaves are prepared and used like spinach, and they are also dried and powdered for use as a condiment.

History of Moringa

It is mostly believed that the moringa tree comes from northern India and was being used in Indian medicine around 5,000 years ago, and there are also accounts of it being made used by the ancient Greeks, Romans, and Egyptians. This tree was, and still is, considered a panacea, and is also called the 'The Magic Tree', 'The Divine Tree', and 'The Miracle Tree' amongst many others. Moringa was used mostly in Ayurveda, where virtually every part was considered useful with a plethora of beneficial attributes. It was hired to support digestion, spleen and eye health, as a cooking additive, and in numerous other ways. Its taste was considered bitter and pungent; its energetic, heating; and its effect upon the dosha (Ayurvedic constitutional type) are balancing to Kapha (dosha ruled by earth and water) and Vata (dosha ruled by air and ether).

The whole tree has been used for erosion control and for building materials to provide shelter. The seed is high in oil, and the fibers remaining after oil extraction are one of the best plant-derived flocculants (clarifying agents) for clarifying water. Further, the roots are believed to taste like horseradish and are thus used as a condiment. Additionally, the flowers are eaten in omelets. The leaves have an extremely high nutrient value and are dried and powdered and put in sauces and baby formula. A beverage is made from the leaf, either as a standard tea or as a type of reconstituted dried leaf juice. In India, the immature seed pods (known as drumsticks) are eaten like asparagus. Further, a nutrient dense formula made from the leaves is sprayed on plants in South America in order to boost corn yields.

Moringa germinates in countries where 5% to 35% of the population is lacking malnutrition. According to an organization working towards feeding malnourished populations known a "Trees for Life "Surprinsinly, moringa germinates in subtropical areas, where malnutrition is generally known. It was as if people had a goldmine in their backyard and simply didn't know it." Many groups are supporting the planting of moringa for personal use in advanced countries, suggesting that each person germinates two or three trees in their backyard thus providing a stable solution to malnutrition and minimized reliance upon imported foods. Moringa has helped in bringing nutrition to these hungry children (and)....it is considered one of the most nutritious vegetables in the world. It is an important nutrient source for nursing mothers as well as growing children.

Nutrients you can find in Moringa

Moringa consist of numerous healthful compounds such as:

- vitamin A
- vitamin B1 (thiamine)
- B2 (riboflavin)
- B3 (niacin), B-6
- folate and ascorbic acid (vitamin C)
- calcium
- potassium
- iron

- magnesium
- phosphorus

Chapter Two

Short Notes on Weight Loss

Weight loss is the process that involve reduction in the accumulation of fats will have gathered in our body over time or some other composition that might have caused weight gain, and this result in slimming down our body stature. Weight loss can be intentional (deliberate action taken to slim down the body stature), such as from **dieting** and **exercise**, or unintentional (unforeseen body reaction that is not triggered by our actions) and it could be as a result of an illness.

Three Things That Build Up Weight Gain in the Body

Weight loss can occur as result of decrease in three (3) compositions in the body that build up to add more weight to our body, and they include;

Body fluid

Water retention in the body can also add weight to the body and this can be cause by so many reasons. A decrease in body fluid can come from the medications you take, lack of fluid intake, fluid loss or it can be as a result an illness such as diabetes.

Muscle mass

Another way you can add weight is by adding up body muscles. Fat is less dense than the muscle (equivalently muscle is more dense than the fat), but occupies less space. This means that you may add muscle and the scale weight increases and find out that you are slimming down. If you can add muscle mass, relaxation of muscle can equally affect weight and causes weight loss

The fats the body as accumulated overtime

The idea of fats in what we consume makes you fat is base on the fact that fats contain more calories comparing to carbohydrates. Overtime when our consumption of fatty foods is high, equally in a short time the fats are stored in our body to build weight in us or add weight to our body. When the fats in the body are decrease, it could be intentional, and this can be probably achieved by the general principle of weight loss such as exercising and dieting.

After pregnancy, it is usual for a woman to lose weight.

Unintetional weight loss

The following causes of weight loss can be referred to as unintentional weight loss, because the actions that propels the reduction in weight wasn't deliberates. The causes include;

- Parasites infection.

- Overactive thyroids

- Depression

- Bowel diseases

- Cancer

- Viral infections, HIV

Chapter Three

Benefits of Moringa

Moringa has the following benefits;

- **Asthma**. Early study shows that using 3 grams of moringa twice daily for 3 weeks decrease the severity of asthma symptoms and effect lung function in adults with mild to moderate asthma.
- **Diabetes**. Early study reveals that using moringa tablets along with a type medicine called sulfonylureas does not effects blood sugar control better than using sulfonylureas alone in people living with diabetes.
- **Increasing breast milk production**. Study regarding the effects of moringa for more breast milk production is conflicting. Some early study reveals that moringa high the milk production, while other early study reveals no importance. An analysis of data from diffrent clinical researches reveals that moringa perfectily increases milk product after a week of use when started on

postpartum day 3. But it's not clear if moringa is useful when taken for longer periods of time.

- **Malnutrition**. Early studies reveals that adding moringa powder to food for 2 months helps improve weight in malnourished children.
- **Menopausal symptoms**. Early research reveals that adding fresh moringa leaves to food for 3 months increase menopausal symptoms such as hot flashes and sleeping problems in healthy, postmenopausal women.
- "Tired blood" (anemia).
- Arthritis.
- As a nutritional supplement.
- Birth control.
- Cancer.
- Constipation.
- Diarrhea.
- Epilepsy.
- Headache.
- Heart problems.
- High blood pressure.
- Increasing sex drive.
- Infections.

- Kidney stones.
- Stomach and intestinal ulcers.
- Stomach pain (gastritis).
- Swelling (inflammation).
- Stimulating immunity.

FAST FACT ON MORINGA

The origin of moringa tree is traced to India but also grows in Asia, Africa and South America.

Moringa contains different kind of protein , vitamins and minerals.

Moringa oleifera has few known side effect.

People taking medication should consult medical personnel before taking moringa.

RISK FACTORS

Some of the medications to be particularly aware of are:

Levothyroxine: Used to fight thyroid problems. Compounds in the moringa leaf may help the thyroid function, but people should not use it in combination with other thyroid medication.

Any medications that might be broken down by the liver: Moringa extract may reduce how fast this happens, which could lead to numerous side effects or complications.

Diabetes medications: Diabetes medications are used to reduce blood sugar, which moringa also does effectively. It is important to ensure blood sugar levels do not get too low.

High blood pressure medication: Moringa has revealed to be active at lowering blood pressure. Taking moringa alongside other drugs that reduce blood pressure may result in it becoming too low.

Chapter Four

Moringa side effects and who should avoid it

The leaf powder had been proved safe in human research, even in larger doses than normal. But you might want to avoid the seed extract consumption, as they have revealed a stage of toxicity in immune cells.

Moringa can have a laxative impact when taken in large quantities or can cause stomach upset, so we decided to start with a small dose—½ to 1 teaspoon per day—to begin.

Moringa is not good for pregnant women to take because of the chemicals possibly discoverd in the root, bark, or flowers of the plant. Taken moringa may cause the uterus to contract or open, possibly leading to a miscarriage or loss of the pregnancy

Interactions with medications

LevothyroxineInteraction Rating: Moderate be cautious with this combination.Contact your medical personnel.

Levothyroxine can be used to reduce thyroid function. Moringa might reduce how much levothyroxine your body take. Consuming moringa along with levothyroxine might reduce the effectiveness of levothyroxine.

Some brands that comprise levothyroxine include Armour Thyroid, Eltroxin, Estre, Euthyrox, Levo-T, Levothroid, Levoxyl, Synthroid, Unithroid, and others.

Some medications are replaced and broken down by the liver. Moringa might reduce how fast the liver breaks down some medications. Consuming moringa along with some medications that are broken down by the liver can high the impacts and side effects of some medications. Before using moringa, contact your medical personnel if you are using any medications that are changed by the liver.

Precaution

Pregnancy: It's not suitable to take the root, bark, or flowers of moringa if you are pregnant. Substances in the root, bark, and flowers might make the uterus contract. In orthodox medicine the root and bark were used for miscarriages. There is not enough information obtainaible concerning the safety of using other parts of moringa during pregnancy. Stay on the safe side and avoid taken it.

Breast-feeding: Moringa is sometimes used to add to breast milk production. It is likely to be safe for the mother when used for several days. But there isn't much information to know if it is good for the nursing infant. Therefore, it is best to stay way from moringa if you are breast-feeding.

Children: Moringa leaf is good when taken by mouth, short-term. Moringa leaf has been tested with apparent and is good in children for up to 2 months.

Chapter Five

Uses of Moringa oleifera as animal feed

Moringa tree has been helpful and important not only to the human beings in terms of their health in one form or the other but also for their livestock (Animal).
Moringa makes a great fodder for cattle. The weight of livestock increased up to 32 per cent through moringa feed. And their milk yield of cows increased by 43 percent.

Policy makers and researchers and others, should organised programs based on creating awareness among local communities and farmers, especially among those who are into livestock production, to emulate the cultivating of moringa as a crop for their livestock. Research Potential of Moringa oleifera as livestock fodder crop.
Moringa as fish food – An alternative plant protein source in fish diet Study, moringa alternative plant protein source in fish diet
And finally a list of conclusions and approval from a study of Moringa diet for rabbits.
Whats good for rabbits must be useful for other animals, right?

Moringa plants are fast-growing and produce high biomass within a short time period when cultivated.
A yield of 616.40 kg/ha dry matter could be obtained at first cut using a planting distance of 1.30 m × 1.30 m.

Moringa leaf meal could be used to changed soyabean meal partially or completely in rabbit diets as a non-conventional protein source, not withstanding the present high cost of the moringa leaf meal. Moringa leaf meal has the potential to produce leaner carcass because of decreased fat deposition in the muscles of rabbits. Moringa leaf meal has the potential to lower cholesterol level in blood and the meat of rabbits. Moringa leaf meal is not poisonous to rabbits at least at the 20% diet inclusion level. Moringa leaf meal diets produced similar economic benefits as soya bean meal diet. Moringa leaf meal could be used to increased daily weight gain, and dry matter and crude protein digestibility of rabbits. Recommendation: Study to support increased in production techniques of the moringa plant is, however, needed to help farmers produce the meal at reduced cost for economic use in animal feeding.

Reseach on Moringa diet for rabbits.

Moringa Oleifera is extremely rich in vital nutrients and, can increase very fast in dry and impoverished areas of the world, where there is scarcity of food. Moringa has gained notoriety as a very nutritious plant that can feed the needy and, in fact, save lives. Moringa leaves or leaf powder can be used successfully as a food supplement to nourish little children, pregnant or nursing women, and of course, anybody else

It is a small effort, a little gesture to give a Moringa seed, but huge effects! Grows a Moringa seed, and it will produce a Moringa tree that increase rapidly and continues to shower you with nutrients for years to come.

Imagine, of all the possibilities the Moringa tree has to offer. A pioneer promoting Moringa oleifera trees, Trees for Life has planted about 200 million Moringa trees in developing countries. We are all grateful for its pioneering actions and vision

Uses and Dosage

The normal dose of moringa is determined by several factors such as the user's age, health, and several other conditions. At this time there is no concrete science evidence to determine an appropriate range of doses for moringa. Have it at the back of your mind that natural products are not always necessarily secure and dosages can be very vital. Be sure to follow relevant directions on product leaflets and consult your medical personnel or doctors or other healthcare professional before using.

Frequently ask question on Moringa

Q: What exactly is moringa?

Moringa is a plant that is originated from the sub-Himalayan areas of India. The leaves, bark, flowers, fruit, seeds, and root are used to make medicine – has been for centuries. Moringa oleifera is arguably the one of the most nutrient-rich plant in the world. Africa Societies and the Middle East have made it a staple of their diets and cuisine for thousands of years and there have been a lot of studies conducted on the plant over the last few decades. It is rich in antioxidants, amino acids, anti-inflammatory properties and many more nutrients and minerals. Because Moringa can be grown cheaply and easily, and the leaves contain lots of vitamins and minerals when dried, moringa is used in India and Africa in feeding programs to combat malnutrition.

Q: Is moringa safe to eat and use?

Absolutely, it's a 100 percent natural plant that has been used for hundreds of generations. In many places, it's one of the few natural food sources denying people from becoming malnourished. It is often called the "Miracle Plant" in these territories. Our Dead Sea Moringa comprises of dried Moringa leaves. The appropriate dose of moringa is determined on several factors such as the user's age, health, and several other conditions. At this time there is no concrete scientific evidence to determine an appropriate range of doses for moringa. Keep in mind that natural products are not always necessarily secured and dosages can be very vital. Be sure to follow relevant directions on product leaflets and consult your medical personnel or doctor or other healthcare professional before using.

Q: Has the moringa in Dead Sea Moringa been genetically modified?

No. The benefits you derived from taking Dead Sea Moringa are the benefits you would gain from eating naturally grown moringa.

Q: How else is moringa used aside from in supplements?

Most parts of the moringa plant are used in food and other substances. The leaves, for example, are commonly used in salads. The seeds can be used to make oil or in other dishes. The plant can also be dried and made into a powder to be used in healthy beverages. The seed cake remaining after oil extraction is used as a fertilizer and also to purify well water and to take out salt from seawater. The immature green pods (drumsticks) are prepared similarly to green beans, while the seeds are removed from more mature pods and cooked like peas or roasted like nuts. The leaves are prepared and used like spinach, and they are also dried and powdered for use as a condiment. However, it's very vital to keep away from eating the root and its extracts.

About the *Author*

Dr. Bayo is a pastor and a medical practioner who studied pharmacy in SefakoMakgatho Health Sciences University (SMU) in South Africa and receive his Phd in Lipscomb University in Missouri-columbia.
He has involved himself into prescriptions and cure of diseases and sickness. He is a solution to many problems amidst its environment such has cancer, stroke infection, erectile dysfuntion, anti-biotic infection, how to reduce your blood pressure and lots more to mention but a little. He has been eagerly and greatly having impact in the life of msny others in the area of pharmaceutical trainings and has been building people to be pharmaceutically awake in order not to be deceived by fake drug sellers out there.

Acknowledgments

My appreciation goes to God, Almighty for the opportunity to collate this manuscript, and for wisdom he gave me to spread the knowledge around. Also I appreciate everyone that supported me during the compilation, proof reading and publishing of the book

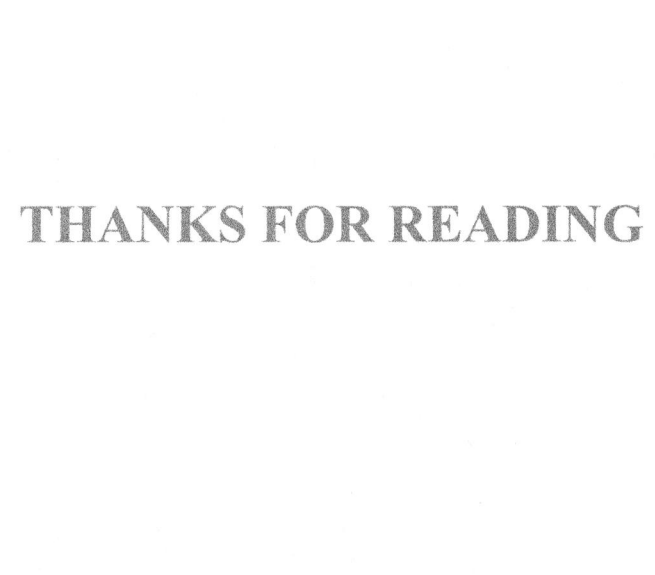
THANKS FOR READING